101 Facts about Hemp CBD Oil

Your Essential Guide to Nature's Remarkable Remedy

By Jake Wood

The information in the following pages is broadly considered to be a truthful and accurate account of facts and as such any inattention, use or misuse of the information in question by the reader will render any resulting actions solely under their purview. There are no scenarios in which the publisher or the original author of this work can be in any fashion deemed liable for any hardship or damages that may befall them after undertaking information described herein.

Additionally, the information in the following pages is intended only for informational purposes and should thus be thought of as universal. As befitting its nature, it is presented without assurance regarding its prolonged validity or interim quality. Trademarks that are mentioned are done without written consent and can in no way be considered an endorsement from the trademark holder.

Table of Contents

Introduction

Congratulations on getting "101 Facts about Hemp CBD Oil"

This ebook is meant to give you as much information on CBD Oil in as short a timeframe as possible. It will try to help you understand what the supplement is and where it comes from. Furthermore it will help you discover why it is used and what the side effects of using the oil may be. It is one of the most comprehensive fun-fact guides on the market to help you understand CBD Oil and how it can benefit you or loved ones.

Chapter 1: What is CBD Oil?

Here are the facts you should be aware of regarding CBD oil and its origins. This information will provide insight into the background of CBD oil, the specific plant components it is derived from, and how these elements impact your body. So, what exactly is CBD oil?

1st fact:
CBD is among over 113 distinct cannabinoid compounds identified in cannabis and hemp plants. Researchers continue to uncover new cannabinoid compounds regularly, suggesting that the list is not yet complete. Many of these compounds are either insignificant or are currently being investigated for

potential applications in contemporary and alternative medicine.

2nd fact:

While CBD is present in cannabis plants, THC is the predominant and most abundant cannabinoid in them. Conversely, THC exists in hemp plants only in minimal quantities, with CBD being the primary, naturally occurring constituent.

3rd fact:

Cannabidiol, or CBD, constitutes up to 40% of the substances extracted from the hemp plant. Other products derived from the plant include hemp oil and hemp seed oil, each serving distinct functions. Hemp seed oil, recognized for its beneficial fatty acid composition, supports healing and is frequently employed to address inflammatory issues and various skin conditions like eczema. In contrast, hemp oil is commonly utilized to produce CBD oil.

4th fact:

Although CBD is a chemical cousin of THC, the psychoactive component in marijuana responsible for the "high," CBD itself is non-addictive. It interacts with our body's internal systems in a non-psychotropic manner, meaning it doesn't induce a high. This crucial characteristic of CBD renders it a safer therapeutic alternative compared to medical marijuana.

5th fact:

In a number of countries, CBD is regarded as a "dietary supplement." As such, when you consume it, you're not actually ingesting something classified as a drug, but instead, you're taking a natural supplement. CBD boasts numerous impressive health advantages, which I will explore further in Chapter 2.

6ᵗʰ fact:

CBD has experienced a surge in popularity in recent times, attributed to its numerous advantages, including alleviating chronic pain and addressing conditions like seizure disorders.

7ᵗʰ fact:

Although CBD oil doesn't induce a high, it does induce substantial alterations in your body. These changes result from cannabinoids binding to your endocannabinoid system, enabling them to modulate functions that help alleviate pain and other challenging or disabling symptoms.

8ᵗʰ fact:

Hemp represents the least processed version of a cannabis plant and notably contains the highest concentration of CBD that can be extracted for its medical advantages, including addressing anxiety, epilepsy, nausea, and cancer.

9ᵗʰ fact:

Although both hemp and marijuana originate from the Cannabis Sativa plant, they are distinct entities with differing genetics, as they are separate strains of the same plant. They are also cultivated for diverse purposes. Historically, and in line with past regulations, hemp has been a legal crop grown to produce fibers for materials like textiles and paper.

On the other hand, marijuana has been prohibited in the majority of countries for an extended period and is generally utilized solely for its psychoactive effects.

10th fact:

Over the years, marijuana cultivators have selectively bred strains to enhance the THC content in their plants. In contrast, hemp farmers have made minimal modifications to their plants. As a result, hemp plants remain exceptionally rich in CBD oil, which is why the majority of CBD oil is sourced from hemp cultivation.

11th fact:

CBD oil is found in hemp oil but not in hemp seed oil. However, the CBD oil typically consumed is a distinct extract in its own right. When CBD oil is extracted for use as a health supplement, it is processed in a way that preserves its purity and eliminates THC and other impurities that could compromise the oil's quality.

12th fact:

The extraction method for CBD oil plays a vital role in preserving the oil's quality. Inefficient extraction can result in inferior CBD oil, diminishing its effectiveness in providing health benefits. The ideal approach for extracting CBD oil involves using carbon dioxide (CO_2) to ensure the oil's integrity is maintained.

13th fact:

A cannabinoid is recognized as the principal chemical compound initially identified in hemp and cannabis plants.

14ᵗʰ fact:

Cannabinoids were first identified in the 1940s when scientists discovered CBD and CBN within the trichomes of the hemp plant. THC was not detected until later, in 1964. For over seven decades, researchers have continued studying the plant, uncovering around 111 additional cannabinoids during that time.

Chapter 2: Why use CBD Oil?

In this chapter, we will delve into the various reasons why you might want to use CBD oil. As the oil was developed to harness its medicinal properties, this chapter will emphasize these benefits, helping you appreciate the true value of this remarkable oil.

15ᵗʰ fact:

In contrast to many traditional medications prescribed for similar purposes, CBD oil does not induce a "high" sensation. Conventional medicines used for the same applications as CBD oil may produce a high or alter an individual's state in a way that makes them feel disconnected from themselves. CBD oil, on the other hand, does not generate these effects. It functions within your body without exerting any psychoactive influence on you.

16ᵗʰ fact:

CBD oil is regarded as beneficial due to its whole-plant nature. Whole-plant medicines have gained increased popularity over time, helping people opt for safer alternatives to traditional medications. Furthermore, since they are derived from whole plants without any added substances, they are thought to be more easily digestible and safer for the body to utilize without causing adverse side effects.

17th fact:

Traditional medications prescribed for the same purposes as CBD oil are often associated with numerous detrimental side effects, some of which can even be life-threatening. In contrast, CBD oil has relatively few side effects. Nonetheless, the potential side effects resulting from CBD oil use will be addressed in "Chapter 5: Potential Adverse Reactions to CBD Oil."

18th fact:

CBD Oil is known to promote emotional homeostasis. This is a state whereby users minimize the ups and downs that are often incurred by emotional upsets, which are known to be common in many ailments, including anything from as simple as chronic pain to as drastic as a terminal illness. Taking a supplement that can support your well-being while also promote your emotional homeostasis means that you will experience less stress. When you experience less stress, not only do you feel better emotionally, but your body also has a stronger chance to fight against anything that may be ailing it. Stress in itself can be an illness. So, no longer having to face these stressors can have a major positive impact on your overall health.

19th fact:

CBD oil is an excellent option for those who are environmentally conscious and seek to prioritize their well-being simultaneously. As previously mentioned, CBD oil is a highly sustainable product derived from a versatile plant with numerous applications. The same plant that yields the medicinal CBD oil also produces fibers utilized in eco-friendly and ethically made textiles and paper products. Consequently, fewer crops need to be cultivated, and the overall impact on the environment is reduced.

20th fact:

Hemp plants reach maturity and are ready for harvest more rapidly than other medicinal plants. This allows for higher yields of hemp from smaller areas of cultivation.

21st fact:

CBD oil is recognized for its antioxidant properties, which can aid your body in neutralizing free radicals. The presence of free radicals in the body has been linked to the development of various diseases and conditions, including cancer. By eliminating them, CBD oil can contribute to promoting long-term overall health and reducing the likelihood of these diseases taking root in your system.

22nd fact:

Owing to its versatile properties, CBD oil can address multiple concerns simultaneously. While you may be using it for a specific purpose, it also works on other symptoms within your body. Consequently, as you find relief from your primary issue, you'll also notice improvements in other areas of your health due to this holistic treatment. CBD oil is among the few remedies that offer numerous positive effects, rather than solely targeting a single condition you're concerned about.

23rd fact:

In contrast to numerous traditional medications, CBD oil can be administered through various methods, allowing you to choose the most suitable and comfortable way to introduce it into your system. This adaptability makes it exceptionally effective in addressing a wide range of ailments, as it can be delivered directly to the source of the symptom swiftly and in the most efficient manner tailored to your preferences.

24th fact:

Rather than relying on over-the-counter medications like ibuprofen and acetaminophen, many medical professionals envision a future where CBD oil becomes a staple supplement in every household. Frequent consumption of the aforementioned drugs has been linked to damage to the stomach lining and worsening symptoms like heartburn and acid reflux. Employing CBD oil as an alternative could potentially be a safer and more effective solution for those seeking relief from issues like headaches or general muscle aches and pains.

25th fact:

CBD oil is recognized for its ability to counterbalance the effects of THC. This is why many recreational marijuana cultivators aim to reduce CBD levels while boosting THC content, as it leads to heightened psychoactive experiences. This also explains why having 0.3% or less THC in your CBD oil is not necessarily detrimental; the CBD will counteract the THC, preventing you from experiencing any psychoactive effects.

26th fact:

While CBD oil is highly regarded for its natural qualities, some individuals might not be able to use it due to potential interactions with medications they are already taking. Additionally, other health-related factors may affect the safety of CBD oil, so it's always advisable to consult your healthcare provider before starting any new supplement. If your practitioner holds conservative views, they might dismiss CBD oil based on their beliefs rather than considering its potential advantages. In such situations, it could be beneficial to seek guidance from a CBD-knowledgeable doctor who can genuinely help you make a decision that aligns with your needs, rather than one influenced by your healthcare practitioner's personal opinions.

27th fact:

CBD oil is a natural plant extract, and in its undiluted form, it can be potentially harmful to the body. That's why CBD oil sellers typically mix it with carrier oils such as fractionated coconut oil or jojoba oil, ensuring its safe application or ingestion without causing adverse side effects. When purchasing CBD oil, it's crucial to thoroughly research the extraction process and the carrier oils used, as these factors can influence the product's quality. It's essential to avoid applying pure CBD oil to your body or ingesting it, as it may lead to severe harm. Like other potent natural extracts, including common essential oils like peppermint or eucalyptus oil, undiluted plant extracts can cause irritation, burns, or other damage when they come into contact with the skin or other body parts.

28th fact:

Certain medications may cause side effects that ironically exacerbate the very symptoms they are intended to alleviate. For instance, some antidepressants can increase depressive symptoms and the likelihood of experiencing suicidal thoughts, placing the user at a heightened risk of suicide. In contrast, CBD oil generally does not have such side effects. The most common issue users may face is the lack of effectiveness or the need to adjust the dosage. As a result, using CBD oil could be a safer option because it minimizes the risk of encountering harmful or potentially fatal side effects.

29th fact:

While CBD oil may not be compatible with all medications, it generally does not interfere with the majority of them. This makes CBD oil a safe alternative to pain medications for alleviating symptoms caused by other medical treatments. It has been particularly popular among cancer patients who may suffer from negative side effects due to aggressive treatments like radiation therapy. Using CBD oil can help reduce these symptoms while still allowing the radiation treatment to effectively carry out its intended purpose.

30th fact:

CBD oil is thought to possess neuroprotective qualities, which means it can help safeguard and support the nervous system. For individuals grappling with neurological disorders like seizures or multiple sclerosis, CBD oil can offer significant relief from the symptoms associated with these conditions.

31st fact:

CBD oil is thought to have beneficial effects on the circulatory system. When consumed in the appropriate dosage, it can help reduce high blood pressure and encourage a healthier functioning heart. The oil's stress- and anxiety-relieving properties are likely responsible for its blood pressure-lowering effects.

32nd fact:

CBD oil is recognized for its potential role in fighting cancer. CBD and other cannabinoids found in the cannabis plant have demonstrated anti-tumor effects and are also known to support conventional treatments. In a recent study, CBD successfully inhibited the growth of various cervical cancer cells. It has also been observed to increase tumor cell death in both colon cancer and leukemia. CBD oil shows promise when used in combination therapies, which are often employed for breast and prostate cancers. Combination therapy means that it can be used alongside other conventional or alternative therapies, working together to help combat tumor growth and cancer cells in patients with various types of cancer.

33rd fact:

Numerous individuals turn to CBD oil for its remarkable pain-relieving properties. This analgesic, a supplement known for easing pain, interacts with receptors in your brain and immune system, helping your body alleviate discomfort and minimize inflammation that may contribute to pain. Thanks to the supplement's nature, these benefits are often experienced without any side effects.

34th fact:

A remarkable and noteworthy aspect of CBD oil is its capacity to reduce or even eliminate seizures in patients who previously experienced numerous episodes. Some manufacturers and distributors of CBD oil have observed patients, who had over 100 seizures per day, experience none for several weeks after using CBD oil. It has even been reported to halt a seizure within minutes of the symptoms starting.

35th fact:

Anxiety is a prevalent issue that affects a significant portion of the population. The Anxiety and Depression Association of America (ADAA) estimates that over 40 million Americans aged 18 and older are impacted by anxiety, which accounts for around 18% of the entire American population. CBD oil has demonstrated promising results in reducing and even eliminating anxiety disorders, even for those who experience debilitating anxiety that prevents them from engaging in everyday activities. CBD oil affects anxiety by calming an individual in their limbic and paralimbic brain areas. Additionally, CBD oil can halt the effects of a panic or anxiety attack within minutes of consumption.

36th fact:

A lesser-known benefit of CBD oil is its potential to help reduce the risk of developing diabetes. A study published in Neuropharmacology demonstrated that CBD oil prevented 67% of non-obese diabetes-prone female mice from developing the disease, while 100% of the untreated mice with the same predisposition went on to develop diabetes. Research is still ongoing to determine the effectiveness of CBD oil in preventing diabetes in adult humans, but the results so far are promising.

37th fact:

A significant number of people in today's society struggle with various sleep-related issues, ranging from restless sleep to full-blown insomnia. One of the effects of CBD oil is its ability to promote better sleep in adults, sometimes causing drowsiness after consumption. This means that instead of relying on potentially addictive and harmful medications that can induce artificial sleep patterns, individuals can opt for a safer alternative through this holistic supplement. CBD oil has been found to encourage healthier and more restful sleep patterns without creating any dependencies or causing harm in any way.

38th fact:

One intriguing benefit many users claim to gain from CBD Oil is its ability to reduce acne. Acne is believed to develop in individuals for various reasons, ranging from genetics to bacteria or even underlying conditions. Recent research has shown that using

CBD Oil through topical application has the potential to improve acne conditions, likely due to its anti-inflammatory effects. Therefore, using CBD Oil can help reduce and alleviate problematic acne in individuals who may be struggling to keep their skin clear and free of blemishes.

39th fact:

CBD Oil has demonstrated antipsychotic properties. Although it is not yet part of standard practice, numerous studies have shown that CBD Oil has the potential to reduce psychotic episodes, such as those associated with schizophrenia or other mental disorders that produce psychotic symptoms. Using this supplement has shown promising benefits in decreasing psychotic symptoms and episodes, helping individuals diagnosed with these types of mental disorders lead a higher quality life, free from the challenging and debilitating symptoms that can hinder them from experiencing a normal life.

40th fact:

Many addiction therapists have been incorporating CBD Oil as a means to help individuals quitting hard drugs like heroin and methamphetamine, in order to alleviate challenging withdrawal symptoms. In studies conducted to investigate the potential benefits of this supplement, researchers have found that CBD Oil can assist individuals struggling with drug addiction in reducing difficult symptoms and preventing dependency and drug-seeking behaviors. In other words, those who were using CBD Oil as part of their treatment were able to go several days or longer without actively seeking out drugs to feed their addiction. This promising finding highlights the potential of CBD Oil in supporting addiction recovery and helping individuals regain control over their lives.

41ˢᵗ fact:

Quitting smoking is another significant benefit of using CBD Oil. Similar to its role in supporting individuals in quitting their addictions to harder drugs, CBD Oil can also aid people in overcoming their addiction to cigarettes. Research studies have demonstrated that individuals who used placebo inhalers experienced no change in their overall cigarette consumption, whereas those who used CBD Oil smoked nearly 40% fewer cigarettes on average each day. This finding suggests that CBD Oil can be a valuable tool in smoking cessation efforts, helping individuals to break free from nicotine addiction and improve their overall health.

42ⁿᵈ fact:

Fibromyalgia is a chronic pain condition with no known cause and few universally effective remedies. It is a somewhat mysterious condition that remains challenging to treat. CBD Oil has shown potential as a powerful pain reliever and symptom management option for those diagnosed with fibromyalgia. In studies conducted, a significant number of participants using CBD Oil treatment experienced reduced symptoms, with some even going on to live symptom-free. While more research is needed, these findings suggest that CBD Oil could be a promising alternative for fibromyalgia patients seeking relief from their symptoms.

43rd fact:

Post-Traumatic Stress Disorder (PTSD) is a complex form of anxiety experienced by individuals who have been exposed to traumatic situations. While PTSD is often associated with war veterans, it can also affect those who have experienced various types of abuse or other traumatic events. CBD Oil has shown promising results in helping individuals with PTSD manage their symptoms. The anti-anxiety, anti-stress, anti-inflammatory, and antipsychotic effects of CBD Oil can provide a more mentally stable environment for those living with PTSD.

By potentially alleviating anxiety, stress, and other PTSD-related symptoms, CBD Oil can support individuals in regaining control over their lives and achieving a better quality of life. However, it is crucial to consult with a healthcare professional before using CBD Oil to manage PTSD, as every individual's needs and circumstances may vary. Further research and clinical trials are needed to fully understand the long-term effects and efficacy of CBD as a treatment for PTSD.

44th fact:

Research and studies on the use of CBD Oil for individuals living with Crohn's disease or irritable bowel syndrome (IBS) have shown promising results. CBD Oil's anti-inflammatory properties and its interaction with the body's endocannabinoid system, which plays a role in gut function, may contribute to the relief of symptoms related to these conditions.

By potentially reducing inflammation in the gastrointestinal tract and modulating gut function,

CBD Oil may help individuals with Crohn's disease or IBS experience less pain, discomfort, and difficulties during bowel movements. However, it is important to note that more research and clinical trials are needed to fully understand the long-term effects and efficacy of CBD as a treatment for these conditions.

45th fact:

Multiple Sclerosis is a chronic and progressive condition that damages the nerves in the brain and spinal cord, resulting in the loss of function in various muscles and body parts. People with this disease often experience difficulty with speech and muscle coordination, as well as blurred vision and extreme fatigue due to the condition. Research indicates that CBD Oil may significantly alleviate symptoms related to this disease, possibly even reversing symptoms and offering protection against the progression of multiple sclerosis. Utilizing CBD Oil could assist individuals with multiple sclerosis in regaining control of their muscles, leading to an improved quality of life after treatment compared to not using CBD Oil.

46th fact:

Rheumatoid arthritis is a painful type of arthritis that causes damage to bones and joints, potentially resulting in deformity over time. CBD Oil, with its anti-inflammatory properties, may help individuals with this condition by reducing symptoms, as inflammation is a primary contributor to the degeneration associated with rheumatoid arthritis. Studies have shown that CBD Oil can decrease joint damage and slow the progression of the disease, enabling those diagnosed with rheumatoid arthritis to enjoy a longer, more fulfilling, and healthier life.

47th fact:

While the research in this area is not as comprehensive, some studies suggest that individuals with broken bones may experience faster healing when using CBD Oil. Bone growth is thought to be one of the potential benefits of this supplement. Ongoing research is being conducted to determine if CBD Oil can contribute to overall improved bone health, which may lead to quicker healing of broken bones and a reduction in the symptomatic side effects associated with osteoporosis.

48th fact:

Psoriasis is a distressing skin condition characterized by extremely dry, flaky skin, causing discomfort for those affected. Topical applications of CBD Oil, such as ointments, creams, serums, or lotions, have been found to help individuals alleviate their psoriasis symptoms and achieve healthier skin. As this condition can be itchy, painful, and cause embarrassment, finding relief from these challenging symptoms can significantly improve the quality of life for those suffering from psoriasis.

49th fact:

Dyskinesia and Restless Leg Syndrome (RLS) are two conditions that cause an involuntary muscle movement in those who are struggling with the conditions. CBD, when combined with a TRPV-1 blocker, has been shown to reduce symptoms of these conditions, supporting individuals in minimizing involuntary muscle movement and thus having greater control over their muscles in general.

50th fact:

Many people suffer from gastrointestinal issues due to poor diets and lifestyle choices, leading to symptoms such as nausea, vomiting, and decreased appetite. CBD Oil has been demonstrated to alleviate these symptoms and assist individuals with poor gut health in regaining their appetite, allowing them to better nourish their bodies. It is worth noting that THC has also been found effective in providing similar benefits. Some medical facilities even prescribe "dronabinol", a medication containing THC, to those who are suffering. However, CBD is gaining more attention for promoting good health over THC, as it is associated with fewer side effects that could impact the patient.

51st fact:

CBD Oil has shown promise in helping individuals with spinal cord injuries, as it can address both nerve damage and the associated pain resulting from such injuries. For those who have experienced traumatic accidents, CBD Oil may offer a non-addictive pain relief option, which can be transformative in their recovery process.

52nd fact:

Researchers are currently exploring the potential benefits of CBD Oil for individuals who have suffered a stroke. Early studies indicate that CBD Oil may be effective in treating and reversing stroke-related symptoms such as nerve damage. Although this research is still in its initial stages, the findings so far have shown promise, with some individuals regaining pain-free control of their limbs and muscles after using CBD Oil as a treatment post-stroke.

Chapter 3: How to use CBD Oil?

Using CBD Oil offers numerous advantages and positive results for those who incorporate it into their routines. You might be curious about the best way to use it. One remarkable aspect of this supplement is its versatility in terms of administration and dosage. Generally, the method of using CBD Oil is contingent on the specific condition being treated. Here are some insights on how to effectively use CBD Oil:

Topical Application

53rd fact:
As a natural plant extract, pure CBD Oil should not be applied topically without first being diluted into a tincture, lotion, balm, or similar product. Applying pure CBD Oil directly onto the skin may lead to irritation, which could negate the therapeutic benefits it is typically known to provide.

54th fact:
The majority of CBD Oil suppliers offer a range of topical CBD Oil products designed for different purposes and with varying dosages. It's always advisable to seek guidance in determining the most

suitable product for your specific needs, especially if you are not already familiar with the options available.

55th fact:
Topical CBD Oil products differ from ingestible CBD Oil products in terms of their effects. They generally work more quickly and provide targeted relief for specific symptoms. For instance, applying CBD Oil topically to an area affected by psoriasis will have a more direct impact on the condition, whereas ingesting it would work throughout the entire body and may take longer to improve the psoriasis symptoms.

56th fact:
Topical CBD Oil application is considered the least invasive method for using CBD Oil. In contrast to ingestion or inhalation, which affect the entire body, topical application primarily focuses on the specific area to which it is applied. Additionally, since CBD Oil in topical products interacts with CB2 receptors near the skin, it activates the endocannabinoid system. This means that, unlike other topical treatments, CBD Oil will not enter your bloodstream through topical products.

57th fact:
Most topical products recommend applying generously, as human skin is known to have a low absorption rate for cannabinoids. This low absorption rate prevents CBD from entering the bloodstream but also means that a larger amount of the product is needed for the skin to absorb enough to experience the desired benefits.

58th fact:

Topical CBD products are not solely for skin-related concerns; they can also be used for joint-related issues and acute pain, such as in cases of rheumatoid arthritis or fibromyalgia. Applying CBD topically directly to the affected area can provide faster relief, making it a more effective option for some of these symptoms compared to ingesting CBD oil.

59th fact:

Individuals with chronic conditions like fibromyalgia might use ingestible CBD oil products to maintain continuous symptom relief, while also applying topical treatments to address any symptom flare-ups that occur despite regular CBD oil use. This combined approach helps provide nearly complete relief from symptoms. This dual treatment can be applied to various conditions that cause pain or other acute physical discomforts.

Ingestion

60th fact:

Ingesting CBD oil is often the simplest method for beginners or children to consume it for symptom relief. This approach is the most frequently recommended for those using CBD oil to address specific conditions. When a CBD oil capsule is swallowed, the concentrated oil passes through the digestive system and is metabolized by the liver, allowing it to enter the bloodstream and start addressing symptoms. This delivery method is similar to how most daily vitamins are absorbed by the body.

61st fact:

Since ingesting CBD oil involves the capsule passing through the digestive system, it can take up to two hours for the full effects to be felt. However, some individuals report noticing positive effects within minutes of consumption. This means that ingesting CBD oil in a concentrated capsule form may provide a slow-release effect, offering symptom relief for up to four hours after taking a single dose.

62nd fact:

For those who would rather not ingest a capsule, CBD Oil is also available in the form of a small tablet that can be placed under the tongue and dissolved by saliva. This method allows the oil to be absorbed directly into the bloodstream, providing faster relief of symptoms that can last for several hours. This can be an ideal option for individuals experiencing sudden and rapidly occurring symptoms, as it bypasses the need to wait for the digestive system to break down the capsule and process the oil.

63rd fact:

An alternative method of consuming CBD Oil is through what is often referred to as "gourmet treats" by dispensaries. These baked goods are infused with CBD Oil, offering the same benefits as other ingestion methods, but without the need to swallow a capsule or dissolve a tablet under the tongue. For some individuals, consuming small portions of CBD-infused foods throughout the day can provide consistent, ongoing effects. Common CBD-infused food items include yogurt, popcorn, cooking oil for salad dressings or as a finishing touch to various dishes, butter, coffee, smoothies, and pasta sauce. With a wide array of edibles available, you can choose the option that suits your preferences and still enjoy the advantages of CBD Oil without resorting to pill form.

64th fact:

When consuming CBD Oil in capsule form, the dosage can be conveniently customized by the dispensary. This allows you to request capsules with lower or higher dosages of CBD Oil, ensuring that you achieve optimal results without overconsumption. Think of these options as similar to "regular strength" and "extra strength" supplements, tailored to suit your individual needs.

65th fact:

Alternative forms of CBD Oil that are neither edibles nor capsules include tinctures and concentrates. These innovative oral products enable CBD Oil to rapidly enter the body's endocannabinoid system, resulting in near-instant effects. Tinctures offer the added benefit of being flavored, making consumption more enjoyable. Concentrates, on the other hand, provide higher dosages and prompt relief from symptoms.

Vaporization

66th fact:

Vaporizing CBD oil is a method of consumption that might cause some people to mistakenly link it with THC or marijuana, believing it can produce a "high." Yet, as outlined in Chapter 1, there are significant differences between CBD oil and marijuana or THC oil. Using vaporized CBD oil will not result in any kind of intoxication unless it contains THC. When vaporizing CBD oil, the same compound is being used, but it is delivered through an alternative method.

67th fact:

Initially, vaporizing CBD oil was among the earliest methods of consumption before extensive research led to the discovery of alternative approaches. Scientists further investigated the plant, aiming to isolate the CBD oil compound and develop new ways to consume the supplement without resorting to vaporization.

68th fact:

Numerous individuals favor vaporizing CBD oil, as it is inhaled into the lungs and swiftly enters the bloodstream along with oxygen. This method offers rapid relief from symptoms that might not respond well to topical applications or could take too long to alleviate through ingestion.

69th fact:

The process of vaporization is not identical to smoking. When a substance is vaporized, it undergoes sufficient heating to transform into steam, through which the CBD compound is transported into the body. In contrast, smoking involves burning the substance to the point of smoke formation, which carries the CBD into the body. While smoke has been linked to cancer-causing effects, vapor has not. This implies that vaporizing CBD Oil avoids wastage and prevents undesirable smoke-related side effects. Individuals with chronic asthma or lung conditions frequently turn to vaporized CBD Oil for immediate relief without the harmful effects of smoking.

70th fact:

To vaporize CBD Oil, it is important to use a concentrated, unadulterated form of the oil. This variety of CBD Oil is typically consumed orally and should not be applied directly to the skin. It is critical to use only pure CBD Oil to avoid inhaling any harmful substances. To prevent any harmful or negative reactions, be sure to inform your dispensary that you plan to vaporize the oil. They can provide you with the appropriate form of oil specifically for vaporizing.

71st fact:

There is a wide variety of vaporizers available in different sizes and shapes. You can choose from pen-style vaporizers that are compact and convenient to carry around, portable vaporizers that are slightly larger but still easily portable, and stationary or desktop vaporizers that are much bigger and can deliver higher doses. Vapor can be obtained through a draw, a tube, a bag, or a balloon, depending on the type of vaporizer. The heating mechanisms in these vaporizers use convection, conduction, or infrared heating to regulate the temperature output, ensuring that the oil is heated to the optimum temperature for vaporization without being burned and producing smoke.

72nd fact:

Certain vaporizers are designed to vaporize dry herbs, which allows your dispensary to provide you with a portion of the cannabis plant that is rich in CBD but has low or negligible levels of THC. To be legal, these supplements must contain less than 0.3% THC. This implies that even if your dispensary provides you with such a supplement, you will not experience any psychoactive effects. Nevertheless, it is crucial to communicate with your dispensary, as some may also provide herbs with high THC levels for other therapeutic purposes.

73rd fact:

Vaporizing remains a popular method for delivering CBD Oil to the body, despite the emergence of other delivery systems. This is because topical creams may require excessive amounts of product to be effective, while ingested CBD Oil can take a longer time to activate. Additionally, vaporizing the oil is much safer than smoking the herb, making it the most secure and efficient approach to deliver CBD into the body.

Chapter 4: Who is CBD Oil for?

In this chapter, we will explore the factors that determine whether a person can safely take CBD Oil or not. It is vital to ensure that CBD Oil is safe for you before consuming it to prevent any potential adverse effects. This is a well-known precautionary measure when starting to use any new supplements or medications.

74th fact:

According to research, most people can safely take CBD Oil without experiencing any significant adverse effects. This supplement is one of the safest and most versatile products available, supporting a range of medical conditions without causing negative side effects in people of different age groups.

75th fact:

CBD Oil is not just beneficial for humans, but it is also being recognized by veterinarians and researchers as a useful supplement for animals. Dogs with epilepsy or senior dogs with arthritis have shown remarkable positive reactions to the supplement, and it has been tested for other ailments in animals with similar positive results. However, it is crucial to note that using other forms of cannabis, including marijuana, is unsafe for animals. Therefore, it is best to seek the assistance of a veterinarian before administering any cannabis-based products to your pets. It is also important to monitor the method of delivery to ensure that it is not harmful to the animal. In this case, the delivery method, rather than the supplement itself, may be harmful to the animal.

Children

76th fact:

Due to the fact that THC and CBD have different

properties, many children can safely consume CBD supplements without experiencing any negative effects. CBD Oil is often used to manage chronic pain and epilepsy in children, among other conditions.

77ᵗʰ fact:

It is important to note that not all CBD Oil products are created equal. Therefore, it is essential to purchase your CBD from a reputable dispensary to ensure that it is safe for consumption. CBD Oil purchased online may contain THC, which is not recommended for children. While CBD does not cause psychoactive effects, THC can be dangerous for children in high amounts. Although the FDA takes steps to eliminate untrustworthy online dealers who sell CBD Oil with higher-than-allowed levels of THC, not all sellers are properly screened and shut down. Therefore, it is crucial to take necessary precautions, especially with children, to avoid any potential adverse reactions.

78ᵗʰ fact:

When it comes to children, seeking advice from a qualified healthcare professional is crucial. While CBD Oil is generally safe and has not been linked to death or any severe long-term effects, giving it to young children may not always be recommended. Some doctors may suggest alternative therapies instead. However, it is essential to discuss your doctor's perspective on CBD Oil and ensure that you fully comprehend their overall position. Some conservative doctors may have moral objections to CBD Oil, resulting in them advising against its use for anyone. Collaborating with a healthcare professional who is knowledgeable about CBD can assist you in making an informed decision.

79th fact:

CBD supplements may help children with conditions such as Autism, Sensory Processing Disorder (SPD), ADD or ADHD, or other challenging disorders to manage their symptoms and feel more integrated into their environment. CBD Oil has been proven to reduce stress levels and promote a sense of belonging, allowing the child to feel more comfortable in their surroundings.

80th fact:

It is essential to note that CBD Oil is not currently legal in all states. Therefore, it is crucial to review the laws of your state and purchase the supplement only when it is legal. Using CBD Oil as an adult in a state where it is illegal can lead to legal repercussions, let alone providing it to a minor. It is crucial to be aware of the laws and abide by them to avoid any potential legal consequences associated with using this supplement.

Adults

81st fact:

CBD Oil can be an expensive medication, but there are ways to find more affordable options. Unfortunately, most healthcare insurance plans do not cover the cost of CBD Oil, so it is an out-of-pocket expense. However, some dispensaries participate in programs that provide discounts or reduced pricing, which can help make the supplement more affordable for those who need it.

82ⁿᵈ fact:

Similar to children, adults who are considering using CBD Oil should seek advice from a healthcare professional. While CBD Oil is generally safe, it is essential to have a qualified practitioner guide you on the proper way to administer it and the appropriate dosage. A knowledgeable healthcare professional can help you find the optimal amount to take, enabling you to experience the benefits without wasting your money or compromising your health.

Seniors

83ʳᵈ fact:

CBD Oil is increasingly being recognized as a safer alternative to traditional medications for seniors experiencing age-related symptoms such as arthritis and pain-related conditions. CBD Oil can offer similar relief from symptoms, without the potential adverse effects associated with other medications, which can be particularly problematic for seniors.

84ᵗʰ fact:

Seniors are more susceptible to developing conditions such as Alzheimer's and Parkinson's disease. CBD Oil is known for its anti-inflammatory and neuroprotective properties, as well as its ability to regulate muscle function and prevent involuntary movement, making it a viable option for relieving symptoms associated with these conditions. These illnesses can cause significant discomfort and disruption to the daily lives of those affected, making it crucial to have effective relief that can improve their overall quality of life.

85th fact:

As seniors age, they often find themselves taking multiple medications, each with its own set of potential side effects. Due to the vulnerability of older bodies, seniors are at a higher risk of experiencing adverse reactions from these medications. In some cases, seniors require additional medications to manage the side effects of their existing medications. Moreover, not all of these medications are covered by insurance, leaving seniors to bear the brunt of exorbitant costs. While CBD Oil may not be a cheaper alternative, it can be comparable in cost per month, and seniors would only need to take one supplement instead of multiple medications. CBD Oil has the potential to improve their quality of life by addressing multiple symptoms, making it a viable option for seniors looking for a simpler, more manageable solution.

86th fact:

While CBD Oil cannot prevent death, it can provide significant relief to individuals suffering from terminal illnesses. For seniors who often face these types of illnesses, incorporating CBD Oil into their treatment plan can greatly improve their quality of life by reducing troublesome symptoms and allowing them to enjoy their later years to the fullest.

87th fact:

As individuals age, they may become increasingly concerned about accidentally taking double doses of medication. CBD Oil can be a reassuring alternative to traditional medications, as it provides similar relief without the danger of accidental overdose. Unlike many medications, CBD Oil does not pose a risk of producing fatal doses, giving seniors peace of mind. However, it is important for seniors to consult with a healthcare practitioner before using CBD Oil to ensure that it is a safe and appropriate option for their individual needs.

CHAPTER 5: POTENTIAL ADVERSE REACTIONS TO CBD OIL

While CBD Oil is generally considered safe and well-tolerated by most individuals, it has been associated with some mild and non-life-threatening side effects in certain cases. Depending on a person's medical condition, CBD Oil may not be a suitable supplement for them. To better understand the potential side effects of CBD Oil, here are some important facts to consider.

Medical Considerations

88th fact:
Individuals who suffer from low blood pressure should avoid taking CBD Oil, as it has the potential to further decrease blood pressure levels, which can lead to cardiac arrest. If you have a history of chronically low blood pressure or have concerns about your heart health, it is advised to avoid the use of CBD Oil.

89th fact:
CBD Oil may react with other medications such as

steroids, HIV antivirals, beta-blockers, antibiotics, calcium channel blockers, NSAIDs, and oral hypoglycemic agents. This interaction can cause negative symptoms and side effects. It is important to inform your doctor about any medications you are taking, even temporarily, and to avoid using CBD Oil in combination with any medication that is deemed unsafe to use with it.

90th fact:

CBD Oil can affect different people differently due to variations in the way they metabolize the supplement. Therefore, it is important to closely monitor individuals who are taking CBD Oil to ensure they are taking the right dosage. Once the correct dosage has been determined, there should be no negative side effects associated with the supplement. Additionally, the symptoms associated with the individual's medical condition should be minimized or eliminated altogether.

91st fact:

Combination therapy is the term used to describe when medications work well together with CBD Oil. It is important to consult with a healthcare professional who has knowledge of CBD Oil to determine if it is safe to use in combination with any current medications. The healthcare professional can also provide guidance on the appropriate dosage and help monitor any potential side effects.

Symptomatic Side Effects

92nd fact:

Although CBD Oil is often used as a treatment for anxiety and depression, some people may actually experience an increase in these symptoms after using the supplement. The reason for this is not fully understood, but it is thought that CBD's ability to slow down certain bodily processes, such as circulation, may trigger feelings of anxiety or depression in some individuals. It is important for people to monitor their symptoms when using CBD Oil and to consult with a healthcare professional if they experience any adverse effects.

93rd fact:

Although CBD Oil should not contain enough THC to have psychoactive effects, some people may still experience symptoms of psychosis after using it. This could be due to a sensitivity to the compound or because they obtained it from a dubious source that contained higher levels of THC than legally permitted. It is crucial to consult a healthcare professional when using CBD Oil and to purchase it from reputable and reliable sources.

94th fact:

Nausea is a common side effect for some people who use CBD Oil, particularly when they take a higher dosage than needed. It could also be due to the concentration of the oil, which may not be suitable for their body. In such cases, individuals may need to consider alternative delivery methods or look for a different supplement or medication that is better suited for their needs.

95th fact:

CBD Oil may cause vomiting in severe cases. This may be due to difficulties in the digestion process or irritation of the stomach lining caused by the oil. If vomiting occurs, stop taking CBD Oil and consult a healthcare practitioner. The practitioner will assess if the dosage is too high or if there is a need to use an alternative method for symptom relief.

96th fact:

CBD Oil is known for its ability to help people get better sleep, which is why it is often used to treat restless sleep or insomnia. However, one of the potential side effects of CBD Oil is drowsiness. If you are not taking CBD Oil for the purpose of improving your sleep and you find that drowsiness is becoming an issue, you may need to adjust your dosage or try a different method of administration to avoid this side effect.

97th fact:

Individuals who consume CBD Oil may experience dry mouth as a side effect. To prevent this, it is recommended to stay hydrated by drinking enough water and sucking on hard candies or cough drops to promote saliva production. If the dry mouth becomes unbearable, adjusting the dosage may help alleviate the symptom.

98th fact:

In some cases, people may experience dizziness after taking CBD Oil. This may be due to a decrease in blood pressure caused by the supplement. To prevent falling or injury, it is important to move slowly and carefully when changing positions. If you experience dizziness, avoid taking any more CBD Oil until you consult with your healthcare practitioner. Continuing to take the supplement despite experiencing low blood pressure can lead to harmful effects.

99th fact:

CBD Oil may cause diarrhea in some individuals, and the exact cause is not fully understood. However, it may be related to digestive system irritation or relaxation. If you experience diarrhea after taking CBD Oil, make sure to stay hydrated by drinking plenty of fluids. If the symptoms persist, consult your doctor to determine whether your dosage should be adjusted or if an alternative method of treatment is necessary.

100th fact:

Individuals who take CBD Oil may experience changes in their appetite. Most commonly, people report an increase in appetite after taking the supplement. However, if you feel a decrease in appetite, this may be an early symptom of nausea. If you feel that your appetite has changed too much and is affecting your health, consult with your doctor to discuss the possibility of adjusting your CBD Oil dosage.

101st fact:

CBD Oil may not be effective in reducing tremors for all individuals with Parkinson's disease. Some people with the condition have noticed increased tremors after taking the supplement, while others experience great relief from their symptoms. It is important to consult with a healthcare practitioner before taking CBD Oil for Parkinson's disease to determine if it is the right choice for your specific case.

Conclusion

Congratulations on completing the comprehensive guide "101 Facts About Hemp CBD Oil"! This guide was created to provide you with a better understanding of CBD Oil and its benefits, as well as its potential drawbacks. CBD Oil has become a popular topic in recent years, and with the government legalizing it, more and more people are interested in using it.

By reading this guide, you should have a better idea of what CBD Oil is, where it comes from, and its uses. Whether you are new to CBD Oil or have been researching it for some time, this guide was designed to be a one-stop source for all your questions.

If you are considering using CBD Oil, it is important to speak with a certified healthcare practitioner who is knowledgeable about CBD Oil. Be sure to disclose any health conditions or medications you are taking to prevent any adverse reactions.

When purchasing CBD Oil, be sure to choose a reputable dispensary that produces safe and high-quality products. Ask them about their production methods and where their products come from to ensure they are trustworthy.

If you found this guide helpful, please consider leaving an honest review on Amazon. Thank you for taking the time to read "101 Facts About Hemp CBD Oil"!

www.ingramcontent.com/pod-product-compliance
Lightning Source LLC
Chambersburg PA
CBHW050707250726

48662CB00002B/887